WORKOUT
LOG

WORKOUT LOG

	S. M.T.W.T.F.S	S. M.T.W.T.F.S	S. M.T.W.T.F.S	S. M.T.W.T.F.S	S. M.T.W.T.F.S	S. M.T.W.T.F.S
Date:						
Weight:						
Hrs of Sleep:						
Warm-up:						

Exercises	lb Weights & Reps	lb Weights & Reps	lb Weights & Reps	lb Weights & Reps	lb Weights & Reps	lb Weights & Reps
Upper Body						
Bench Press						
Bicep Curls						
Tricep Curls						
Overhead Press						
Lat Pulldown						
Upperhand Rows						
Abs						
Lower Body						
Deadlift						
Leg Press						
Squat						
Leg Curl						
Calf Extensions						
Abs						
Cardio						
Time						
Distance						
Intensity						
Spinning						

Notes:

_____

_____

_____

_____

WORKOUT LOG

	S. M.T.W.T.F.S	S. M.T.W.T.F.S	S. M.T.W.T.F.S	S. M.T.W.T.F.S	S. M.T.W.T.F.S	S. M.T.W.T.F.S
Date:						
Weight:						
Hrs of Sleep:						
Warm-up:						

Exercises	lb Weights & Reps	lb Weights & Reps	lb Weights & Reps	lb Weights & Reps	lb Weights & Reps	lb Weights & Reps
Upper Body						
Bench Press						
Bicep Curls						
Tricep Curls						
Overhead Press						
Lat Pulldown						
Upperhand Rows						
Abs						
Lower Body						
Deadlift						
Leg Press						
Squat						
Leg Curl						
Calf Extensions						
Abs						
Cardio						
Time						
Distance						
Intensity						
Spinning						

Notes:

_____

_____

_____

_____

WORKOUT LOG

	S. M.T.W.T.F.S	S. M.T.W.T.F.S	S. M.T.W.T.F.S	S. M.T.W.T.F.S	S. M.T.W.T.F.S	S. M.T.W.T.F.S
Date:						
Weight:						
Hrs of Sleep:						
Warm-up:						

Exercises	lb Weights & Reps	lb Weights & Reps	lb Weights & Reps	lb Weights & Reps	lb Weights & Reps	lb Weights & Reps
Upper Body						
Bench Press						
Bicep Curls						
Tricep Curls						
Overhead Press						
Lat Pulldown						
Upperhand Rows						
Abs						
Lower Body						
Deadlift						
Leg Press						
Squat						
Leg Curl						
Calf Extensions						
Abs						
Cardio						
Time						
Distance						
Intensity						
Spinning						

Notes:

_____

_____

_____

_____

WORKOUT LOG

	S. M.T.W.T.F.S	S. M.T.W.T.F.S	S. M.T.W.T.F.S	S. M.T.W.T.F.S	S. M.T.W.T.F.S	S. M.T.W.T.F.S
Date:						
Weight:						
Hrs of Sleep:						
Warm-up:						

Exercises	lb Weights & Reps	lb Weights & Reps	lb Weights & Reps	lb Weights & Reps	lb Weights & Reps	lb Weights & Reps
Upper Body						
Bench Press						
Bicep Curls						
Tricep Curls						
Overhead Press						
Lat Pulldown						
Upperhand Rows						
Abs						
Lower Body						
Deadlift						
Leg Press						
Squat						
Leg Curl						
Calf Extensions						
Abs						
Cardio						
Time						
Distance						
Intensity						
Spinning						

Notes:

_____

_____

_____

_____

WORKOUT LOG

	S. M.T.W.T.F.S	S. M.T.W.T.F.S	S. M.T.W.T.F.S	S. M.T.W.T.F.S	S. M.T.W.T.F.S	S. M.T.W.T.F.S
Date:						
Weight:						
Hrs of Sleep:						
Warm-up:						

Exercises	lb Weights & Reps	lb Weights & Reps	lb Weights & Reps	lb Weights & Reps	lb Weights & Reps	lb Weights & Reps
Upper Body						
Bench Press						
Bicep Curls						
Tricep Curls						
Overhead Press						
Lat Pulldown						
Upperhand Rows						
Abs						
Lower Body						
Deadlift						
Leg Press						
Squat						
Leg Curl						
Calf Extensions						
Abs						
Cardio						
Time						
Distance						
Intensity						
Spinning						

Notes:

_____

_____

_____

_____

WORKOUT LOG

	S. M.T.W.T.F.S	S. M.T.W.T.F.S	S. M.T.W.T.F.S	S. M.T.W.T.F.S	S. M.T.W.T.F.S	S. M.T.W.T.F.S
Date:						
Weight:						
Hrs of Sleep:						
Warm-up:						

Exercises	lb Weights & Reps	lb Weights & Reps	lb Weights & Reps	lb Weights & Reps	lb Weights & Reps	lb Weights & Reps
Upper Body						
Bench Press						
Bicep Curls						
Tricep Curls						
Overhead Press						
Lat Pulldown						
Upperhand Rows						
Abs						
Lower Body						
Deadlift						
Leg Press						
Squat						
Leg Curl						
Calf Extensions						
Abs						
Cardio						
Time						
Distance						
Intensity						
Spinning						

Notes:

_____

_____

_____

_____

WORKOUT LOG

	S. M.T.W.T.F.S	S. M.T.W.T.F.S	S. M.T.W.T.F.S	S. M.T.W.T.F.S	S. M.T.W.T.F.S	S. M.T.W.T.F.S
Date:						
Weight:						
Hrs of Sleep:						
Warm-up:						

Exercises	lb Weights & Reps	lb Weights & Reps	lb Weights & Reps	lb Weights & Reps	lb Weights & Reps	lb Weights & Reps
Upper Body						
Bench Press						
Bicep Curls						
Tricep Curls						
Overhead Press						
Lat Pulldown						
Upperhand Rows						
Abs						
Lower Body						
Deadlift						
Leg Press						
Squat						
Leg Curl						
Calf Extensions						
Abs						
Cardio						
Time						
Distance						
Intensity						
Spinning						

Notes:

_____

_____

_____

_____

WORKOUT LOG

	S. M.T.W.T.F.S	S. M.T.W.T.F.S	S. M.T.W.T.F.S	S. M.T.W.T.F.S	S. M.T.W.T.F.S	S. M.T.W.T.F.S
Date:						
Weight:						
Hrs of Sleep:						
Warm-up:						

Exercises	lb Weights & Reps	lb Weights & Reps	lb Weights & Reps	lb Weights & Reps	lb Weights & Reps	lb Weights & Reps
Upper Body						
Bench Press						
Bicep Curls						
Tricep Curls						
Overhead Press						
Lat Pulldown						
Upperhand Rows						
Abs						
Lower Body						
Deadlift						
Leg Press						
Squat						
Leg Curl						
Calf Extensions						
Abs						
Cardio						
Time						
Distance						
Intensity						
Spinning						

Notes:

_____

_____

_____

_____

WORKOUT LOG

	S. M.T.W.T.F.S	S. M.T.W.T.F.S	S. M.T.W.T.F.S	S. M.T.W.T.F.S	S. M.T.W.T.F.S	S. M.T.W.T.F.S
Date:						
Weight:						
Hrs of Sleep:						
Warm-up:						

Exercises	lb Weights & Reps	lb Weights & Reps	lb Weights & Reps	lb Weights & Reps	lb Weights & Reps	lb Weights & Reps
Upper Body						
Bench Press						
Bicep Curls						
Tricep Curls						
Overhead Press						
Lat Pulldown						
Upperhand Rows						
Abs						
Lower Body						
Deadlift						
Leg Press						
Squat						
Leg Curl						
Calf Extensions						
Abs						
Cardio						
Time						
Distance						
Intensity						
Spinning						

Notes:

_____

_____

_____

_____

WORKOUT LOG

	S.M.T.W.T.F.S	S.M.T.W.T.F.S	S.M.T.W.T.F.S	S.M.T.W.T.F.S	S.M.T.W.T.F.S	S.M.T.W.T.F.S
Date:						
Weight:						
Hrs of Sleep:						
Warm-up:						

Exercises	lb Weights & Reps	lb Weights & Reps	lb Weights & Reps	lb Weights & Reps	lb Weights & Reps	lb Weights & Reps
Upper Body						
Bench Press						
Bicep Curls						
Tricep Curls						
Overhead Press						
Lat Pulldown						
Upperhand Rows						
Abs						
Lower Body						
Deadlift						
Leg Press						
Squat						
Leg Curl						
Calf Extensions						
Abs						
Cardio						
Time						
Distance						
Intensity						
Spinning						

Notes:

_____

_____

_____

_____

_____

WORKOUT LOG

Exercises	S. M.T.W.T.F.S	S. M.T.W.T.F.S	S. M.T.W.T.F.S	S. M.T.W.T.F.S	S. M.T.W.T.F.S	S. M.T.W.T.F.S
Date:						
Weight:						
Hrs of Sleep:						
Warm-up:						

Exercises	lb Weights & Reps	lb Weights & Reps	lb Weights & Reps	lb Weights & Reps	lb Weights & Reps	lb Weights & Reps
Upper Body						
Bench Press						
Bicep Curls						
Tricep Curls						
Overhead Press						
Lat Pulldown						
Upperhand Rows						
Abs						
Lower Body						
Deadlift						
Leg Press						
Squat						
Leg Curl						
Calf Extensions						
Abs						
Cardio						
Time						
Distance						
Intensity						
Spinning						

Notes:

_____

_____

_____

_____

WORKOUT LOG

Exercises	S.M.T.W.T.F.S	S.M.T.W.T.F.S	S.M.T.W.T.F.S	S.M.T.W.T.F.S	S.M.T.W.T.F.S	S.M.T.W.T.F.S
Date:						
Weight:						
Hrs of Sleep:						
Warm-up:						

Exercises	lb Weights & Reps	lb Weights & Reps	lb Weights & Reps	lb Weights & Reps	lb Weights & Reps	lb Weights & Reps
Upper Body						
Bench Press						
Bicep Curls						
Tricep Curls						
Overhead Press						
Lat Pulldown						
Upperhand Rows						
Abs						
Lower Body						
Deadlift						
Leg Press						
Squat						
Leg Curl						
Calf Extensions						
Abs						
Cardio						
Time						
Distance						
Intensity						
Spinning						

Notes:

_____

_____

_____

_____

WORKOUT LOG

	S. M.T.W.T.F.S	S. M.T.W.T.F.S	S. M.T.W.T.F.S	S. M.T.W.T.F.S	S. M.T.W.T.F.S	S. M.T.W.T.F.S
Date:						
Weight:						
Hrs of Sleep:						
Warm-up:						

Exercises	lb Weights & Reps	lb Weights & Reps	lb Weights & Reps	lb Weights & Reps	lb Weights & Reps	lb Weights & Reps
Upper Body						
Bench Press						
Bicep Curls						
Tricep Curls						
Overhead Press						
Lat Pulldown						
Upperhand Rows						
Abs						
Lower Body						
Deadlift						
Leg Press						
Squat						
Leg Curl						
Calf Extensions						
Abs						
Cardio						
Time						
Distance						
Intensity						
Spinning						

Notes:
_____
_____
_____
_____

WORKOUT LOG

	S. M.T.W.T.F.S	S. M.T.W.T.F.S	S. M.T.W.T.F.S	S. M.T.W.T.F.S	S. M.T.W.T.F.S	S. M.T.W.T.F.S
Date:						
Weight:						
Hrs of Sleep:						
Warm-up:						

Exercises	lb Weights & Reps	lb Weights & Reps	lb Weights & Reps	lb Weights & Reps	lb Weights & Reps	lb Weights & Reps
Upper Body						
Bench Press						
Bicep Curls						
Tricep Curls						
Overhead Press						
Lat Pulldown						
Upperhand Rows						
Abs						
Lower Body						
Deadlift						
Leg Press						
Squat						
Leg Curl						
Calf Extensions						
Abs						
Cardio						
Time						
Distance						
Intensity						
Spinning						

Notes:

_____

_____

_____

_____

WORKOUT LOG

	S. M.T.W.T.F.S	S. M.T.W.T.F.S	S. M.T.W.T.F.S	S. M.T.W.T.F.S	S. M.T.W.T.F.S	S. M.T.W.T.F.S
Date:						
Weight:						
Hrs of Sleep:						
Warm-up:						

Exercises	lb Weights & Reps	lb Weights & Reps	lb Weights & Reps	lb Weights & Reps	lb Weights & Reps	lb Weights & Reps
Upper Body						
Bench Press						
Bicep Curls						
Tricep Curls						
Overhead Press						
Lat Pulldown						
Upperhand Rows						
Abs						
Lower Body						
Deadlift						
Leg Press						
Squat						
Leg Curl						
Calf Extensions						
Abs						
Cardio						
Time						
Distance						
Intensity						
Spinning						

Notes:

_____

_____

_____

_____

_____

WORKOUT LOG

	S. M.T.W.T.F.S	S. M.T.W.T.F.S	S. M.T.W.T.F.S	S. M.T.W.T.F.S	S. M.T.W.T.F.S	S. M.T.W.T.F.S
Date:						

Weight: _____

Hrs of Sleep: _____

Warm-up: _____

Exercises	lb Weights & Reps	lb Weights & Reps	lb Weights & Reps	lb Weights & Reps	lb Weights & Reps	lb Weights & Reps
Upper Body						
Bench Press						
Bicep Curls						
Tricep Curls						
Overhead Press						
Lat Pulldown						
Upperhand Rows						
Abs						
Lower Body						
Deadlift						
Leg Press						
Squat						
Leg Curl						
Calf Extensions						
Abs						
Cardio						
Time						
Distance						
Intensity						
Spinning						

Notes:

_____

_____

_____

_____

WORKOUT LOG

	S. M.T.W.T.F.S	S. M.T.W.T.F.S	S. M.T.W.T.F.S	S. M.T.W.T.F.S	S. M.T.W.T.F.S	S. M.T.W.T.F.S
Date:						
Weight:						
Hrs of Sleep:						
Warm-up:						

Exercises	lb Weights & Reps	lb Weights & Reps	lb Weights & Reps	lb Weights & Reps	lb Weights & Reps	lb Weights & Reps
Upper Body						
Bench Press						
Bicep Curls						
Tricep Curls						
Overhead Press						
Lat Pulldown						
Upperhand Rows						
Abs						
Lower Body						
Deadlift						
Leg Press						
Squat						
Leg Curl						
Calf Extensions						
Abs						
Cardio						
Time						
Distance						
Intensity						
Spinning						

Notes:

_____

_____

_____

_____

WORKOUT LOG

	S. M.T.W.T.F.S	S. M.T.W.T.F.S	S. M.T.W.T.F.S	S. M.T.W.T.F.S	S. M.T.W.T.F.S	S. M.T.W.T.F.S
Date:						
Weight:						
Hrs of Sleep:						
Warm-up:						

Exercises	lb Weights & Reps	lb Weights & Reps	lb Weights & Reps	lb Weights & Reps	lb Weights & Reps	lb Weights & Reps
Upper Body						
Bench Press						
Bicep Curls						
Tricep Curls						
Overhead Press						
Lat Pulldown						
Upperhand Rows						
Abs						
Lower Body						
Deadlift						
Leg Press						
Squat						
Leg Curl						
Calf Extensions						
Abs						
Cardio						
Time						
Distance						
Intensity						
Spinning						

Notes:
_____
_____
_____
_____

WORKOUT LOG

	S. M.T.W.T.F.S	S. M.T.W.T.F.S	S. M.T.W.T.F.S	S. M.T.W.T.F.S	S. M.T.W.T.F.S	S. M.T.W.T.F.S
Date:						
Weight:						
Hrs of Sleep:						
Warm-up:						

Exercises	lb Weights & Reps	lb Weights & Reps	lb Weights & Reps	lb Weights & Reps	lb Weights & Reps	lb Weights & Reps
Upper Body						
Bench Press						
Bicep Curls						
Tricep Curls						
Overhead Press						
Lat Pulldown						
Upperhand Rows						
Abs						
Lower Body						
Deadlift						
Leg Press						
Squat						
Leg Curl						
Calf Extensions						
Abs						
Cardio						
Time						
Distance						
Intensity						
Spinning						

Notes:

_____

_____

_____

_____

WORKOUT LOG

	S. M.T.W.T.F.S	S. M.T.W.T.F.S	S. M.T.W.T.F.S	S. M.T.W.T.F.S	S. M.T.W.T.F.S	S. M.T.W.T.F.S
Date:						
Weight:						
Hrs of Sleep:						
Warm-up:						

Exercises	lb Weights & Reps	lb Weights & Reps	lb Weights & Reps	lb Weights & Reps	lb Weights & Reps	lb Weights & Reps
Upper Body						
Bench Press						
Bicep Curls						
Tricep Curls						
Overhead Press						
Lat Pulldown						
Upperhand Rows						
Abs						
Lower Body						
Deadlift						
Leg Press						
Squat						
Leg Curl						
Calf Extensions						
Abs						
Cardio						
Time						
Distance						
Intensity						
Spinning						

Notes:

_____

_____

_____

_____

WORKOUT LOG

	S. M.T.W.T.F.S	S. M.T.W.T.F.S	S. M.T.W.T.F.S	S. M.T.W.T.F.S	S. M.T.W.T.F.S	S. M.T.W.T.F.S
Date:						
Weight:						
Hrs of Sleep:						
Warm-up:						

Exercises	lb Weights & Reps	lb Weights & Reps	lb Weights & Reps	lb Weights & Reps	lb Weights & Reps	lb Weights & Reps
Upper Body						
Bench Press						
Bicep Curls						
Tricep Curls						
Overhead Press						
Lat Pulldown						
Upperhand Rows						
Abs						
Lower Body						
Deadlift						
Leg Press						
Squat						
Leg Curl						
Calf Extensions						
Abs						
Cardio						
Time						
Distance						
Intensity						
Spinning						

Notes:

_____

_____

_____

_____

WORKOUT LOG

	S. M. T. W. T. F. S	S. M. T. W. T. F. S	S. M. T. W. T. F. S	S. M. T. W. T. F. S	S. M. T. W. T. F. S	S. M. T. W. T. F. S
Date:						
Weight:						
Hrs of Sleep:						
Warm-up:						

Exercises	lb Weights & Reps	lb Weights & Reps	lb Weights & Reps	lb Weights & Reps	lb Weights & Reps	lb Weights & Reps
Upper Body						
Bench Press						
Bicep Curls						
Tricep Curls						
Overhead Press						
Lat Pulldown						
Upperhand Rows						
Abs						
Lower Body						
Deadlift						
Leg Press						
Squat						
Leg Curl						
Calf Extensions						
Abs						
Cardio						
Time						
Distance						
Intensity						
Spinning						

Notes:

_____

_____

_____

_____

WORKOUT LOG

	S. M.T.W.T.F.S	S. M.T.W.T.F.S	S. M.T.W.T.F.S	S. M.T.W.T.F.S	S. M.T.W.T.F.S	S. M.T.W.T.F.S
Date:						
Weight:						
Hrs of Sleep:						
Warm-up:						

Exercises	lb Weights & Reps	lb Weights & Reps	lb Weights & Reps	lb Weights & Reps	lb Weights & Reps	lb Weights & Reps
Upper Body						
Bench Press						
Bicep Curls						
Tricep Curls						
Overhead Press						
Lat Pulldown						
Upperhand Rows						
Abs						
Lower Body						
Deadlift						
Leg Press						
Squat						
Leg Curl						
Calf Extensions						
Abs						
Cardio						
Time						
Distance						
Intensity						
Spinning						

Notes:

_____

_____

_____

_____

WORKOUT LOG

	S. M.T.W.T.F.S	S. M.T.W.T.F.S	S. M.T.W.T.F.S	S. M.T.W.T.F.S	S. M.T.W.T.F.S	S. M.T.W.T.F.S
Date:						
Weight:						
Hrs of Sleep:						
Warm-up:						

Exercises	lb Weights & Reps	lb Weights & Reps	lb Weights & Reps	lb Weights & Reps	lb Weights & Reps	lb Weights & Reps
Upper Body						
Bench Press						
Bicep Curls						
Tricep Curls						
Overhead Press						
Lat Pulldown						
Upperhand Rows						
Abs						
Lower Body						
Deadlift						
Leg Press						
Squat						
Leg Curl						
Calf Extensions						
Abs						
Cardio						
Time						
Distance						
Intensity						
Spinning						

Notes:

_____

_____

_____

_____

WORKOUT LOG

	S. M.T.W.T.F.S	S. M.T.W.T.F.S	S. M.T.W.T.F.S	S. M.T.W.T.F.S	S. M.T.W.T.F.S	S. M.T.W.T.F.S
Date:						
Weight:						
Hrs of Sleep:						
Warm-up:						

Exercises	lb Weights & Reps	lb Weights & Reps	lb Weights & Reps	lb Weights & Reps	lb Weights & Reps	lb Weights & Reps
Upper Body						
Bench Press						
Bicep Curls						
Tricep Curls						
Overhead Press						
Lat Pulldown						
Upperhand Rows						
Abs						
Lower Body						
Deadlift						
Leg Press						
Squat						
Leg Curl						
Calf Extensions						
Abs						
Cardio						
Time						
Distance						
Intensity						
Spinning						

Notes:

_____

_____

_____

_____

WORKOUT LOG

	S. M.T.W.T.F.S	S. M.T.W.T.F.S	S. M.T.W.T.F.S	S. M.T.W.T.F.S	S. M.T.W.T.F.S	S. M.T.W.T.F.S
Date:						
Weight:						
Hrs of Sleep:						
Warm-up:						

Exercises	lb Weights & Reps	lb Weights & Reps	lb Weights & Reps	lb Weights & Reps	lb Weights & Reps	lb Weights & Reps
Upper Body						
Bench Press						
Bicep Curls						
Tricep Curls						
Overhead Press						
Lat Pulldown						
Upperhand Rows						
Abs						
Lower Body						
Deadlift						
Leg Press						
Squat						
Leg Curl						
Calf Extensions						
Abs						
Cardio						
Time						
Distance						
Intensity						
Spinning						

Notes:

_____

_____

_____

_____

WORKOUT LOG

	S. M.T.W.T.F.S	S. M.T.W.T.F.S	S. M.T.W.T.F.S	S. M.T.W.T.F.S	S. M.T.W.T.F.S	S. M.T.W.T.F.S
Date:						

Weight: _____

Hrs of Sleep: _____

Warm-up: _____

Exercises	lb Weights & Reps	lb Weights & Reps	lb Weights & Reps	lb Weights & Reps	lb Weights & Reps	lb Weights & Reps
Upper Body						
Bench Press						
Bicep Curls						
Tricep Curls						
Overhead Press						
Lat Pulldown						
Upperhand Rows						
Abs						
Lower Body						
Deadlift						
Leg Press						
Squat						
Leg Curl						
Calf Extensions						
Abs						
Cardio						
Time						
Distance						
Intensity						
Spinning						

Notes:

_____

_____

_____

_____

WORKOUT LOG

	S. M.T.W.T.F.S	S. M.T.W.T.F.S	S. M.T.W.T.F.S	S. M.T.W.T.F.S	S. M.T.W.T.F.S	S. M.T.W.T.F.S
Date:						

Weight: _____

Hrs of Sleep: _____

Warm-up: _____

Exercises	lb Weights & Reps	lb Weights & Reps	lb Weights & Reps	lb Weights & Reps	lb Weights & Reps	lb Weights & Reps
Upper Body						
Bench Press						
Bicep Curls						
Tricep Curls						
Overhead Press						
Lat Pulldown						
Upperhand Rows						
Abs						
Lower Body						
Deadlift						
Leg Press						
Squat						
Leg Curl						
Calf Extensions						
Abs						
Cardio						
Time						
Distance						
Intensity						
Spinning						

Notes:

_____

_____

_____

_____

WORKOUT LOG

	S. M.T.W.T.F.S	S. M.T.W.T.F.S	S. M.T.W.T.F.S	S. M.T.W.T.F.S	S. M.T.W.T.F.S	S. M.T.W.T.F.S
Date:						
Weight:						
Hrs of Sleep:						
Warm-up:						

Exercises	lb Weights & Reps	lb Weights & Reps	lb Weights & Reps	lb Weights & Reps	lb Weights & Reps	lb Weights & Reps
Upper Body						
Bench Press						
Bicep Curls						
Tricep Curls						
Overhead Press						
Lat Pulldown						
Upperhand Rows						
Abs						
Lower Body						
Deadlift						
Leg Press						
Squat						
Leg Curl						
Calf Extensions						
Abs						
Cardio						
Time						
Distance						
Intensity						
Spinning						

Notes:

_____

_____

_____

_____

WORKOUT LOG

	S. M.T.W.T.F.S	S. M.T.W.T.F.S	S. M.T.W.T.F.S	S. M.T.W.T.F.S	S. M.T.W.T.F.S	S. M.T.W.T.F.S
Date:						
Weight:						
Hrs of Sleep:						
Warm-up:						

Exercises	lb Weights & Reps	lb Weights & Reps	lb Weights & Reps	lb Weights & Reps	lb Weights & Reps	lb Weights & Reps
Upper Body						
Bench Press						
Bicep Curls						
Tricep Curls						
Overhead Press						
Lat Pulldown						
Upperhand Rows						
Abs						
Lower Body						
Deadlift						
Leg Press						
Squat						
Leg Curl						
Calf Extensions						
Abs						
Cardio						
Time						
Distance						
Intensity						
Spinning						

Notes:

_____

_____

_____

_____

WORKOUT LOG

	S. M.T.W.T.F.S	S. M.T.W.T.F.S	S. M.T.W.T.F.S	S. M.T.W.T.F.S	S. M.T.W.T.F.S	S. M.T.W.T.F.S
Date:						
Weight:						
Hrs of Sleep:						
Warm-up:						

Exercises	lb Weights & Reps	lb Weights & Reps	lb Weights & Reps	lb Weights & Reps	lb Weights & Reps	lb Weights & Reps
Upper Body						
Bench Press						
Bicep Curls						
Tricep Curls						
Overhead Press						
Lat Pulldown						
Upperhand Rows						
Abs						
Lower Body						
Deadlift						
Leg Press						
Squat						
Leg Curl						
Calf Extensions						
Abs						
Cardio						
Time						
Distance						
Intensity						
Spinning						

Notes:

_____
_____
_____
_____

WORKOUT LOG

	S. M.T.W.T.F.S	S. M.T.W.T.F.S	S. M.T.W.T.F.S	S. M.T.W.T.F.S	S. M.T.W.T.F.S	S. M.T.W.T.F.S
Date:						

Weight: _____

Hrs of Sleep: _____

Warm-up: _____

Exercises	lb Weights & Reps	lb Weights & Reps	lb Weights & Reps	lb Weights & Reps	lb Weights & Reps	lb Weights & Reps
Upper Body						
Bench Press						
Bicep Curls						
Tricep Curls						
Overhead Press						
Lat Pulldown						
Upperhand Rows						
Abs						
Lower Body						
Deadlift						
Leg Press						
Squat						
Leg Curl						
Calf Extensions						
Abs						
Cardio						
Time						
Distance						
Intensity						
Spinning						

Notes:

_____

_____

_____

_____

WORKOUT LOG

	S. M.T.W.T.F.S	S. M.T.W.T.F.S	S. M.T.W.T.F.S	S. M.T.W.T.F.S	S. M.T.W.T.F.S	S. M.T.W.T.F.S
Date:						
Weight:						
Hrs of Sleep:						
Warm-up:						

Exercises	lb Weights & Reps	lb Weights & Reps	lb Weights & Reps	lb Weights & Reps	lb Weights & Reps	lb Weights & Reps
Upper Body						
Bench Press						
Bicep Curls						
Tricep Curls						
Overhead Press						
Lat Pulldown						
Upperhand Rows						
Abs						
Lower Body						
Deadlift						
Leg Press						
Squat						
Leg Curl						
Calf Extensions						
Abs						
Cardio						
Time						
Distance						
Intensity						
Spinning						

Notes:

_____

_____

_____

_____

WORKOUT LOG

	S.M.T.W.T.F.S	S.M.T.W.T.F.S	S.M.T.W.T.F.S	S.M.T.W.T.F.S	S.M.T.W.T.F.S	S.M.T.W.T.F.S
Date:						
Weight:						
Hrs of Sleep:						
Warm-up:						

Exercises	lb Weights & Reps	lb Weights & Reps	lb Weights & Reps	lb Weights & Reps	lb Weights & Reps	lb Weights & Reps
Upper Body						
Bench Press						
Bicep Curls						
Tricep Curls						
Overhead Press						
Lat Pulldown						
Upperhand Rows						
Abs						
Lower Body						
Deadlift						
Leg Press						
Squat						
Leg Curl						
Calf Extensions						
Abs						
Cardio						
Time						
Distance						
Intensity						
Spinning						

Notes:

_____

_____

_____

_____

_____

WORKOUT LOG

	S. M.T.W.T.F.S	S. M.T.W.T.F.S	S. M.T.W.T.F.S	S. M.T.W.T.F.S	S. M.T.W.T.F.S	S. M.T.W.T.F.S
Date:						
Weight:						
Hrs of Sleep:						
Warm-up:						

Exercises	lb Weights & Reps	lb Weights & Reps	lb Weights & Reps	lb Weights & Reps	lb Weights & Reps	lb Weights & Reps
Upper Body						
Bench Press						
Bicep Curls						
Tricep Curls						
Overhead Press						
Lat Pulldown						
Upperhand Rows						
Abs						
Lower Body						
Deadlift						
Leg Press						
Squat						
Leg Curl						
Calf Extensions						
Abs						
Cardio						
Time						
Distance						
Intensity						
Spinning						

Notes:

_____

_____

_____

_____

WORKOUT LOG

	S. M.T.W.T.F.S	S. M.T.W.T.F.S	S. M.T.W.T.F.S	S. M.T.W.T.F.S	S. M.T.W.T.F.S	S. M.T.W.T.F.S
Date:						
Weight:						
Hrs of Sleep:						
Warm-up:						

Exercises	lb Weights & Reps	lb Weights & Reps	lb Weights & Reps	lb Weights & Reps	lb Weights & Reps	lb Weights & Reps
Upper Body						
Bench Press						
Bicep Curls						
Tricep Curls						
Overhead Press						
Lat Pulldown						
Upperhand Rows						
Abs						
Lower Body						
Deadlift						
Leg Press						
Squat						
Leg Curl						
Calf Extensions						
Abs						
Cardio						
Time						
Distance						
Intensity						
Spinning						

Notes:

WORKOUT LOG

Exercises	S. M.T.W.T.F.S	S. M.T.W.T.F.S	S. M.T.W.T.F.S	S. M.T.W.T.F.S	S. M.T.W.T.F.S	S. M.T.W.T.F.S
Date:						
Weight:						
Hrs of Sleep:						
Warm-up:						

Exercises	lb Weights & Reps	lb Weights & Reps	lb Weights & Reps	lb Weights & Reps	lb Weights & Reps	lb Weights & Reps
Upper Body						
Bench Press						
Bicep Curls						
Tricep Curls						
Overhead Press						
Lat Pulldown						
Upperhand Rows						
Abs						
Lower Body						
Deadlift						
Leg Press						
Squat						
Leg Curl						
Calf Extensions						
Abs						
Cardio						
Time						
Distance						
Intensity						
Spinning						

Notes:

_____

_____

_____

_____

WORKOUT LOG

	S.M.T.W.T.F.S	S.M.T.W.T.F.S	S.M.T.W.T.F.S	S.M.T.W.T.F.S	S.M.T.W.T.F.S	S.M.T.W.T.F.S
Date:						
Weight:						
Hrs of Sleep:						
Warm-up:						

Exercises	lb Weights & Reps	lb Weights & Reps	lb Weights & Reps	lb Weights & Reps	lb Weights & Reps	lb Weights & Reps
Upper Body						
Bench Press						
Bicep Curls						
Tricep Curls						
Overhead Press						
Lat Pulldown						
Upperhand Rows						
Abs						
Lower Body						
Deadlift						
Leg Press						
Squat						
Leg Curl						
Calf Extensions						
Abs						
Cardio						
Time						
Distance						
Intensity						
Spinning						

Notes:

_____

_____

_____

_____

WORKOUT LOG

	S. M.T.W.T.F.S	S. M.T.W.T.F.S	S. M.T.W.T.F.S	S. M.T.W.T.F.S	S. M.T.W.T.F.S	S. M.T.W.T.F.S
Date:						
Weight:						
Hrs of Sleep:						
Warm-up:						

Exercises	lb Weights & Reps	lb Weights & Reps	lb Weights & Reps	lb Weights & Reps	lb Weights & Reps	lb Weights & Reps
Upper Body						
Bench Press						
Bicep Curls						
Tricep Curls						
Overhead Press						
Lat Pulldown						
Upperhand Rows						
Abs						
Lower Body						
Deadlift						
Leg Press						
Squat						
Leg Curl						
Calf Extensions						
Abs						
Cardio						
Time						
Distance						
Intensity						
Spinning						

Notes:

_____

_____

_____

_____

WORKOUT LOG

	S. M.T.W.T.F.S	S. M.T.W.T.F.S	S. M.T.W.T.F.S	S. M.T.W.T.F.S	S. M.T.W.T.F.S	S. M.T.W.T.F.S
Date:						
Weight:						
Hrs of Sleep:						
Warm-up:						

Exercises	lb Weights & Reps	lb Weights & Reps	lb Weights & Reps	lb Weights & Reps	lb Weights & Reps	lb Weights & Reps
Upper Body						
Bench Press						
Bicep Curls						
Tricep Curls						
Overhead Press						
Lat Pulldown						
Upperhand Rows						
Abs						
Lower Body						
Deadlift						
Leg Press						
Squat						
Leg Curl						
Calf Extensions						
Abs						
Cardio						
Time						
Distance						
Intensity						
Spinning						

Notes:

_____

_____

_____

_____

_____

WORKOUT LOG

	S.M.T.W.T.F.S	S.M.T.W.T.F.S	S.M.T.W.T.F.S	S.M.T.W.T.F.S	S.M.T.W.T.F.S	S.M.T.W.T.F.S
Date:						
Weight:						
Hrs of Sleep:						
Warm-up:						

Exercises	lb Weights & Reps	lb Weights & Reps	lb Weights & Reps	lb Weights & Reps	lb Weights & Reps	lb Weights & Reps
Upper Body						
Bench Press						
Bicep Curls						
Tricep Curls						
Overhead Press						
Lat Pulldown						
Upperhand Rows						
Abs						
Lower Body						
Deadlift						
Leg Press						
Squat						
Leg Curl						
Calf Extensions						
Abs						
Cardio						
Time						
Distance						
Intensity						
Spinning						

Notes:

WORKOUT LOG

	S. M.T.W.T.F.S	S. M.T.W.T.F.S	S. M.T.W.T.F.S	S. M.T.W.T.F.S	S. M.T.W.T.F.S	S. M.T.W.T.F.S
Date:						
Weight:						
Hrs of Sleep:						
Warm-up:						

Exercises	lb Weights & Reps	lb Weights & Reps	lb Weights & Reps	lb Weights & Reps	lb Weights & Reps	lb Weights & Reps
Upper Body						
Bench Press						
Bicep Curls						
Tricep Curls						
Overhead Press						
Lat Pulldown						
Upperhand Rows						
Abs						
Lower Body						
Deadlift						
Leg Press						
Squat						
Leg Curl						
Calf Extensions						
Abs						
Cardio						
Time						
Distance						
Intensity						
Spinning						

Notes:

_____

_____

_____

_____

WORKOUT LOG

	S. M.T.W.T.F.S	S. M.T.W.T.F.S	S. M.T.W.T.F.S	S. M.T.W.T.F.S	S. M.T.W.T.F.S	S. M.T.W.T.F.S
Date:						
Weight:						
Hrs of Sleep:						
Warm-up:						

Exercises	lb Weights & Reps	lb Weights & Reps	lb Weights & Reps	lb Weights & Reps	lb Weights & Reps	lb Weights & Reps
Upper Body						
Bench Press						
Bicep Curls						
Tricep Curls						
Overhead Press						
Lat Pulldown						
Upperhand Rows						
Abs						
Lower Body						
Deadlift						
Leg Press						
Squat						
Leg Curl						
Calf Extensions						
Abs						
Cardio						
Time						
Distance						
Intensity						
Spinning						

Notes:

_____

_____

_____

_____

WORKOUT LOG

	S. M.T.W.T.F.S	S. M.T.W.T.F.S	S. M.T.W.T.F.S	S. M.T.W.T.F.S	S. M.T.W.T.F.S	S. M.T.W.T.F.S
Date:						

Weight: _____

Hrs of Sleep: _____

Warm-up: _____

Exercises	lb Weights & Reps	lb Weights & Reps	lb Weights & Reps	lb Weights & Reps	lb Weights & Reps	lb Weights & Reps
Upper Body						
Bench Press						
Bicep Curls						
Tricep Curls						
Overhead Press						
Lat Pulldown						
Upperhand Rows						
Abs						
Lower Body						
Deadlift						
Leg Press						
Squat						
Leg Curl						
Calf Extensions						
Abs						
Cardio						
Time						
Distance						
Intensity						
Spinning						

Notes:

_____

_____

_____

_____

WORKOUT LOG

	S.M.T.W.T.F.S	S.M.T.W.T.F.S	S.M.T.W.T.F.S	S.M.T.W.T.F.S	S.M.T.W.T.F.S	S.M.T.W.T.F.S
Date:						
Weight:						
Hrs of Sleep:						
Warm-up:						

Exercises	lb Weights & Reps	lb Weights & Reps	lb Weights & Reps	lb Weights & Reps	lb Weights & Reps	lb Weights & Reps
Upper Body						
Bench Press						
Bicep Curls						
Tricep Curls						
Overhead Press						
Lat Pulldown						
Upperhand Rows						
Abs						
Lower Body						
Deadlift						
Leg Press						
Squat						
Leg Curl						
Calf Extensions						
Abs						
Cardio						
Time						
Distance						
Intensity						
Spinning						

Notes:
_____
_____
_____
_____

WORKOUT LOG

Exercises	S.M.T.W.T.F.S	S.M.T.W.T.F.S	S.M.T.W.T.F.S	S.M.T.W.T.F.S	S.M.T.W.T.F.S	S.M.T.W.T.F.S
Date:						
Weight:						
Hrs of Sleep:						
Warm-up:						

Exercises	lb Weights & Reps	lb Weights & Reps	lb Weights & Reps	lb Weights & Reps	lb Weights & Reps	lb Weights & Reps
Upper Body						
Bench Press						
Bicep Curls						
Tricep Curls						
Overhead Press						
Lat Pulldown						
Upperhand Rows						
Abs						
Lower Body						
Deadlift						
Leg Press						
Squat						
Leg Curl						
Calf Extensions						
Abs						
Cardio						
Time						
Distance						
Intensity						
Spinning						

Notes:

_____

_____

_____

_____

_____

WORKOUT LOG

	S. M.T.W.T.F.S	S. M.T.W.T.F.S	S. M.T.W.T.F.S	S. M.T.W.T.F.S	S. M.T.W.T.F.S	S. M.T.W.T.F.S
Date:						
Weight:						
Hrs of Sleep:						
Warm-up:						

Exercises	lb Weights & Reps	lb Weights & Reps	lb Weights & Reps	lb Weights & Reps	lb Weights & Reps	lb Weights & Reps
Upper Body						
Bench Press						
Bicep Curls						
Tricep Curls						
Overhead Press						
Lat Pulldown						
Upperhand Rows						
Abs						
Lower Body						
Deadlift						
Leg Press						
Squat						
Leg Curl						
Calf Extensions						
Abs						
Cardio						
Time						
Distance						
Intensity						
Spinning						

Notes:

_____

_____

_____

_____

WORKOUT LOG

	S. M.T.W.T.F.S	S. M.T.W.T.F.S	S. M.T.W.T.F.S	S. M.T.W.T.F.S	S. M.T.W.T.F.S	S. M.T.W.T.F.S
Date:						
Weight:						
Hrs of Sleep:						
Warm-up:						

Exercises	lb Weights & Reps	lb Weights & Reps	lb Weights & Reps	lb Weights & Reps	lb Weights & Reps	lb Weights & Reps
Upper Body						
Bench Press						
Bicep Curls						
Tricep Curls						
Overhead Press						
Lat Pulldown						
Upperhand Rows						
Abs						
Lower Body						
Deadlift						
Leg Press						
Squat						
Leg Curl						
Calf Extensions						
Abs						
Cardio						
Time						
Distance						
Intensity						
Spinning						

Notes:

_____

_____

_____

_____

WORKOUT LOG

	S. M.T.W.T.F.S	S. M.T.W.T.F.S	S. M.T.W.T.F.S	S. M.T.W.T.F.S	S. M.T.W.T.F.S	S. M.T.W.T.F.S
Date:						
Weight:						
Hrs of Sleep:						
Warm-up:						

Exercises	lb Weights & Reps	lb Weights & Reps	lb Weights & Reps	lb Weights & Reps	lb Weights & Reps	lb Weights & Reps
Upper Body						
Bench Press						
Bicep Curls						
Tricep Curls						
Overhead Press						
Lat Pulldown						
Upperhand Rows						
Abs						
Lower Body						
Deadlift						
Leg Press						
Squat						
Leg Curl						
Calf Extensions						
Abs						
Cardio						
Time						
Distance						
Intensity						
Spinning						

Notes:

_____

_____

_____

_____

WORKOUT LOG

	S. M.T.W.T.F.S	S. M.T.W.T.F.S	S. M.T.W.T.F.S	S. M.T.W.T.F.S	S. M.T.W.T.F.S	S. M.T.W.T.F.S
Date:						
Weight:						
Hrs of Sleep:						
Warm-up:						

Exercises	lb Weights & Reps	lb Weights & Reps	lb Weights & Reps	lb Weights & Reps	lb Weights & Reps	lb Weights & Reps
Upper Body						
Bench Press						
Bicep Curls						
Tricep Curls						
Overhead Press						
Lat Pulldown						
Upperhand Rows						
Abs						
Lower Body						
Deadlift						
Leg Press						
Squat						
Leg Curl						
Calf Extensions						
Abs						
Cardio						
Time						
Distance						
Intensity						
Spinning						

Notes:

_____

_____

_____

_____

WORKOUT LOG

	S. M.T.W.T.F.S	S. M.T.W.T.F.S	S. M.T.W.T.F.S	S. M.T.W.T.F.S	S. M.T.W.T.F.S	S. M.T.W.T.F.S
Date:						
Weight:						
Hrs of Sleep:						
Warm-up:						

Exercises	lb Weights & Reps	lb Weights & Reps	lb Weights & Reps	lb Weights & Reps	lb Weights & Reps	lb Weights & Reps
Upper Body						
Bench Press						
Bicep Curls						
Tricep Curls						
Overhead Press						
Lat Pulldown						
Upperhand Rows						
Abs						
Lower Body						
Deadlift						
Leg Press						
Squat						
Leg Curl						
Calf Extensions						
Abs						
Cardio						
Time						
Distance						
Intensity						
Spinning						

Notes:

_____

_____

_____

_____

WORKOUT LOG

Exercises	S. M.T.W.T.F.S	S. M.T.W.T.F.S	S. M.T.W.T.F.S	S. M.T.W.T.F.S	S. M.T.W.T.F.S	S. M.T.W.T.F.S
Date:						
Weight:						
Hrs of Sleep:						
Warm-up:						
	lb Weights & Reps	lb Weights & Reps	lb Weights & Reps	lb Weights & Reps	lb Weights & Reps	lb Weights & Reps
Upper Body						
Bench Press						
Bicep Curls						
Tricep Curls						
Overhead Press						
Lat Pulldown						
Upperhand Rows						
Abs						
Lower Body						
Deadlift						
Leg Press						
Squat						
Leg Curl						
Calf Extensions						
Abs						
Cardio						
Time						
Distance						
Intensity						
Spinning						

Notes:

_____

_____

_____

_____

WORKOUT LOG

	S. M.T.W.T.F.S	S. M.T.W.T.F.S	S. M.T.W.T.F.S	S. M.T.W.T.F.S	S. M.T.W.T.F.S	S. M.T.W.T.F.S
Date:						
Weight:						
Hrs of Sleep:						
Warm-up:						

Exercises	lb Weights & Reps	lb Weights & Reps	lb Weights & Reps	lb Weights & Reps	lb Weights & Reps	lb Weights & Reps
Upper Body						
Bench Press						
Bicep Curls						
Tricep Curls						
Overhead Press						
Lat Pulldown						
Upperhand Rows						
Abs						
Lower Body						
Deadlift						
Leg Press						
Squat						
Leg Curl						
Calf Extensions						
Abs						
Cardio						
Time						
Distance						
Intensity						
Spinning						

Notes:

_____

_____

_____

_____

WORKOUT LOG

Exercises	S.M.T.W.T.F.S	S.M.T.W.T.F.S	S.M.T.W.T.F.S	S.M.T.W.T.F.S	S.M.T.W.T.F.S	S.M.T.W.T.F.S
Date:						
Weight:						
Hrs of Sleep:						
Warm-up:						

Exercises	lb Weights & Reps	lb Weights & Reps	lb Weights & Reps	lb Weights & Reps	lb Weights & Reps	lb Weights & Reps
Upper Body						
Bench Press						
Bicep Curls						
Tricep Curls						
Overhead Press						
Lat Pulldown						
Upperhand Rows						
Abs						
Lower Body						
Deadlift						
Leg Press						
Squat						
Leg Curl						
Calf Extensions						
Abs						
Cardio						
Time						
Distance						
Intensity						
Spinning						

Notes:

_____

_____

_____

_____

WORKOUT LOG

Exercises	S. M.T.W.T.F.S lb Weights & Reps	S. M.T.W.T.F.S lb Weights & Reps	S. M.T.W.T.F.S lb Weights & Reps	S. M.T.W.T.F.S lb Weights & Reps	S. M.T.W.T.F.S lb Weights & Reps	S. M.T.W.T.F.S lb Weights & Reps
Date:						
Weight:						
Hrs of Sleep:						
Warm-up:						
Upper Body						
Bench Press						
Bicep Curls						
Tricep Curls						
Overhead Press						
Lat Pulldown						
Upperhand Rows						
Abs						
Lower Body						
Deadlift						
Leg Press						
Squat						
Leg Curl						
Calf Extensions						
Abs						
Cardio						
Time						
Distance						
Intensity						
Spinning						

Notes:

_____

_____

_____

_____

_____

www.ingramcontent.com/pod-product-compliance
Lightning Source LLC
Chambersburg PA
CBHW081422280526
45788CB00009B/3197

9 781542 602136